# Contents

**Foreword** *vi*

1 **Prevalence** *1*

2 **Economic burden of the disease** *3*

3 **The problem of underdiagnosis** *5*
COPD screening criteria *6*

4 **Initial evaluation** *7*
Diagnosis and initial assessment *7*

5 **Follow-up** *8*
Factors to be considered during COPD follow-up *8*
Scheduled visits *9*

6 **Spirometry** *10*
Bronchodilator test assessment *10*
Preparation for forced spirometry *11*
Forced spirometry manoeuvre *11*
Forced spirometry evaluation *12*

7 **Algorithm for COPD diagnosis** *13*
COPD initial assessment *13*
COPD additional tests *13*
COPD optional tests *15*

8 **Classification of severity** *16*
Severity classification of COPD (GOLD Guidelines) *16*

9 **Causes of COPD** *17*
Tobacco smoking *17*
*Air pollutants* *17*
*Alpha-1 antitrypsin deficiency* *18*
COPD aetiology *18*

10 **Smoking cessation** 19
Initial evaluation and smoking cessation follow-up 19
*Therapies for smoking cessation* 19

11 **Pharmacological treatment of COPD** 22
Objectives of treatment of COPD 22
Stable COPD main thresholds treatment 23
*Vaccination* 23
*Bronchodilator treatment* 23
*Dosage, posology and administration route of main inhaled bronchodilator drugs* 24
*Beta-2 adrenergics (short acting)* 25
*Beta-2 adrenergics (long acting)* 25
*Anticholinergics (short and long acting)* 25
*Methylxanthines* 25
Anti-inflammatory treatment 26
*Oral corticosteroids and COPD* 26
*Inhaled corticosteroids* 26
*Adverse effects of COPD treatment* 28
Stepwise treatment 28
*Proposal of treatment (mild and moderate COPD)* 29
*Proposal of treatment (severe COPD)* 29
Oxygen therapy 29
*Long term oxygen therapy indication* 30
Inhalation devices 30
*Advantages of inhaled therapy* 30
Metered-dose inhalers (MDI) 31
*Pressurized cartridge* 31
*Autohaler systems* 31
*Inhalation chambers* 31
Dry powder inhalers 31
*Turbuhaler* 32
*Accuhaler* 32

# Management Of Chronic Obstructive Pulmonary Disease

## A Pocket Guide

Coordinator

**Marc Miravitlles MD**
Consultant Chest Physician
Pneumology Department
Clinic Institut of Pneumology and Thoracic Surgery (IDIBAPS)
Hospital Clínic
Barcelona, Spain

Authors

**Cristian de la Roza MD**
Researcher, Chest Physician
Pneumology Department
Clinic Institut of Pneumology and Thoracic Surgery (IDIBAPS)
Hospital Clínic
Barcelona, Spain

**Beatriz Lara MD**
Researcher, Chest Physician
Pneumology Department
Clinic Institut of Pneumology and Thoracic Surgery (IDIBAPS)
Hospital Clínic
Barcelona, Spain

**Sara Vilà MD**
Researcher, Chest Physician
Pneumology Department
Clinic Institut of Pneumology and Thoracic Surgery (IDIBAPS)
Hospital Clínic
Barcelona, Spain

*Current Medical Literature*

The editors and publishers have undertaken reasonable steps to ensure that the information contained in this publication is correct at the time of printing. These steps have included checking the information against generally accepted sources and submitting the publication to peer review.

Despite these steps, the editors and publishers cannot guarantee that the information is or will remain correct and complete. The sources which they have used and the peer review process are by no means infallible. Developments in medical and/or clinical knowledge may show, or suggest, that some or all of the information is incorrect, incomplete or misleading.

Accordingly, neither the editors nor the publisher nor any other person involved in the production of this publication can accept any legal responsibility for any loss or damage caused by the use of any of the information contained in this publication, except when that loss and damage has been caused by their own negligence.

Since there is a possibility that the information contained in this publication may be incorrect, incomplete or misleading, and the consequences of acting upon information which is incorrect, incomplete or misleading could be very serious, readers are strongly advised to take steps to verify the information contained in this publication prior to using it. Before using information relating to any drug or piece of medical equipment, particularly those which are new and/or unfamiliar, it is essential that readers consult the most recent version of the drug or equipment manufacturer's product literature to verify that the information is both accurate and up-to-date.

Published by

Current Medical Literature Ltd
40-42 Osnaburgh Street
London NW1 3ND, UK

Fax: +44 (0) 20 7465 8380
Tel: +44 (0) 20 7465 8377
E-mail: philip.shaw@currentmedicalliterature.com



Editor: Philip Shaw
Production Manager: Danielle Underwood

ISBN: 1-85009-225-7

Printed in Italy

*HandiHaler* 32
*Main characteristics of the different devices* 32

12 **Non-pharmacological treatment** 33
Rehabilitation 33
*Exercise training* 33
*Respiratory physiotherapy* 33
*Nutrition counselling* 33
*Education* 34
Surgical treatments 34
*Lung volume reduction surgery (LVRS)* 34
*Transplantation* 35
Conclusions 36

13 **Acute exacerbations** 37
Definition 37
Incidence and importance 37
*Risk factors for failure after ambulatory treatment of exacerbation of COPD* 37
*Risk factors for hospitalization for exacerbation of COPD* 38
*Risk factors for frequent exacerbations of COPD (> 2 per year)* 39
Aetiology 39
*Aetiology of acute exacerbations of COPD* 40
Treatment: antibiotics 40
*Factors influencing antibiotic choice for exacerbations of COPD* 41
Treatment: bronchodilators and corticosteroids 42

14 **When to refer a COPD patient to hospital or a specialist** 45
Criteria for referral to pneumologist 45
Indications for arterial gasometry 45
Factors suggesting good COPD management 46

**Bibliography** 47

# Foreword

Clinicians generally do a good job diagnosing and managing patients with hypertension, diabetes, and several other chronic disorders. They generally do a poor job of diagnosing and managing COPD. Why the difference, and is it important?

First, why the difference? Awareness of many chronic conditions, such as hypertension and diabetes, has increased enormously over the past few decades, in large part due to extensive research into outcomes of treated and untreated disease. As the science base for the benefits of tight control of chronic conditions such as hypertension and diabetes has grown, so have the large-scale educational programs aimed at both clinicians and the lay public. In turn, as the knowledge of the medical profession and the lay public has increased in relation to such chronic diseases, so have the expectations and accountability increased. Our patients expect to have their blood pressure measured. We comply and treat abnormal findings. In part as a consequence of this increased awareness, expectation and accountability, cardiovascular mortality has steadily decreased over the past decade, at least in the US where the public health education programs have been particularly effective.

COPD poses a challenge. It is often viewed as a disease that is self-inflicted, affects older adults, is irreversible and difficult to treat, and is more of a nuisance than an important public health problem. Consequently it is under-diagnosed, under-appreciated and under-treated.

Next, is it important? Returning to the analogy of hypertension, there is general acceptance of the value of treating hypertension aggressively. Cardiovascular disease is the leading cause of morbidity and mortality in developed countries. It erodes quality of life and is very costly. It is eminently treatable and treatment is relatively inexpensive and effective. COPD, on the other hand, is viewed as an irreversible disease, hard to treat, and costly because it often leads to intensive use of health care resources (hospitalization, emergency visits and long-term oxygen). Lack of awareness of its impact and importance, and its treatability, often leads to it being ignored by primary care clinicians, at least until it is advanced.

As laid out superbly in this compact monograph, COPD is on the increase in most countries. It affects 8% or more of the population over age 50 years in most developed countries. It is very costly. Until recently, it was considered a disease that affected men, and women were generally spared. Now, the statistics are strikingly different: the prevalence of COPD in adult women and men is now approximately equal in the US, the country with arguably the best population-based data on prevalence based on lung function. This is, of course, largely a consequence of women adopting smoking in equal numbers as men. This alarming situation is much the same in most developed countries where women have sought, and achieved, the opportunity to adopt the same lifestyle as their male counterparts.

# Foreword

The message for primary care practitioners is clear: COPD is worth diagnosing and can be managed so that the quality of life of patients with COPD can be greatly improved, and mortality decreased. It can also be prevented. The public health messages are that cough and sputum are not normal, and that shortness of breath is not an inevitable part of ageing. Practitioners should look for COPD, especially in all of their patients who smoke or have respiratory symptoms; they should have access to spirometry, and should treat patients with COPD actively. And perhaps of greatest importance, we need to change our thinking from one of pessimism (COPD is an irreversible disease) to one of optimism (active management of COPD can greatly improve quality of life). This is a challenge for us all but one that will bring great rewards if we are able to meet it.

A. Sonia Buist M.D.
Professor of Medicine
Pulmonary & Critical Care Medicine
Oregon Health & Science University
Portland, OR, USA

# Prevalence

1 (i)

Chronic obstructive pulmonary disease (COPD) is a frequent cause of morbidity and mortality in developed countries. It is the fourth leading cause of chronic morbidity and mortality in the USA. Despite the campaigns against tobacco smoking, prevalence of the disease and mortality rates due to COPD continue to increase and COPD is considered the only preventable disease that is still on the increase in developed countries. Age-adjusted mortality rate increased 47.3% in the USA from 1979 to 1993.

Several studies have shown significant differences in COPD prevalence among different countries. Although much of this difference can be attributed to smoking habits, environmental factors and diagnostic or coding practices, it may also reflect biological or genetic differences in the risk of obstructive lung disease.

In Spain, 9% of adults between the ages of 40 and 70 suffer from COPD, although only 22% are diagnosed. A UK study found a prevalence of COPD in the general population aged between 60 and 75 years to be 9.9%, with 52% of the cases not been previously diagnosed. Chronic airflow obstruction prevalence of 9.5% and 8.6%, in men and women respectively, between the ages of 40 and 59 in Denmark has been reported, and the figures were 4.5% and 4.8%, respectively, in Norway in the same age group.

Chronic bronchitis with or without airflow obstruction is even more frequent. A recent European survey in young adults aged between 20 and 44 has observed a mean prevalence of 2.6%, ranging from 0.7% to 9.7%. The mean percentage of current smokers in this age group was 40%.

Since smoking is, by far, the main risk factor for the development of COPD, it is possible to estimate the number of people suffering from some degree of chronic airflow limitation based in prevalence of current and former smokers. Most of these patients remain undiagnosed with mild forms of the disease, but they can potentially progress to more severe COPD.

| Country | % Smoking rate for people >45 years of age (ever smoked) | People with COPD |
|---|---|---|
| UK | 60 | 2 960 000 |
| Germany | 22 | 2 661 000 |
| Italy | 47 | 2 637 000 |
| France | 33 | 2 633 000 |
| Spain | 50 | 1 517 000 |
| USA | 70 | 15 337 000 |

(adapted from Stang et al 1999)

# 1 (ii) Prevalence

The occurrence of undiagnosed COPD has been recognized in all developed countries. Reasons for the delay in diagnosis include the slow progression of the disease, the self-inflicted nature of COPD, with patients being reluctant to seek medical attention, and the lack of awareness of COPD and its related morbidity and mortality by general physicians.

COPD has been classically a men's disease, but prevalence in women has increased in recent years due to the increasing number of women older than 50 smoking. In the USA, statistics have shown that, for the first time, mortality due to COPD in women was equal to that in men in 2000.

# Economic burden of the disease

2 (i)

Costs due to chronic diseases can be divided into direct medical costs (derived directly from the medical attention to the patient, such as drugs, medical visits, hospitalization, rehabilitation, etc) and indirect costs (loss of productivity due to absence from work and disability pensions). Indirect costs are more difficult to calculate, and may vary greatly from country to country due to different health services. Direct medical costs are thus more suitable for comparisons between countries.

COPD is a frequent cause of hospitalizations, disability and death, and generates a great social and economic burden. The economic impact of COPD in 1993 was estimated to be more than $15.5 billion in the USA, with $6.1 billion for hospitalization. In Spain, a recent study has shown that the mean direct medical cost of a COPD patient followed up in primary care was €1880, with mean cost of the severe disease almost double that of the mild disease. According to the prevalence of the disease and the number of diagnosed patients in the country, global direct cost of COPD was calculated to be €510.52 million or €13.82 per capita. To put this into perspective, a recent study in the Netherlands obtained a cost for asthma and COPD of $23 per capita.

The most important component of direct costs for COPD is hospitalization, which represents approximately 40–50% of all costs. Drug acquisition costs range from 30–45% and clinic visits and diagnostic tests represent between 10–20% of all costs.

# 2 (ii) Economic burden of the disease

| Country | Costs evaluated | Cost per patient/year | Global cost/year | Reference |
|---|---|---|---|---|
| USA | Direct | Stage I = $1681<br>Stage II= $5037<br>Stage III= $10 812 | | Hilleman et al, 2000 |
| Sweden | Direct and Indirect | | Direct $111 M<br>Indirect $173 M | Jacobson et al, 2000 |
| USA | Direct | Emphysema $1341<br>Chronic bronchitis $816 | $14 500 M | Wilson et al, 2000 |
| Netherlands | Direct | $876 | | Rutten van Mölken et al, 2000 |
| Sweden | Direct and Indirect | Stage I = $792<br>Stage II = $4101<br>Stage III = $10 334 | Direct plus Indirect $871 M | Jansson et al, 2002 |
| Italy | Direct | Stage I = €151<br>Stage II = €3001<br>Stage III = €3912 | | Dal Negro et al, 2002 |
| Spain | Direct | Stage I= €1510<br>Stage II= €2104<br>Stage III= €2988 | €510 M | Miravitlles et al, 2003 |

$ = US dollars, € = Euros, M = millions, Global cost = cost estimated for the whole country

Since patients with severe disease are those that incur higher medical costs, it is financially crucial to diagnose COPD at an early stage. Early detection of COPD among smoking adults may permit the implementation of smoking cessation strategies and other appropriate treatment.

# The problem of underdiagnosis

3 (i)

Patients at early stage COPD are either unaware of their condition or reluctant to consult their physician for respiratory symptoms. Consequently, most mild cases do not receive active counselling against tobacco smoking or appropriate pharmacological treatment. Moreover, some treatments administered to patients with COPD are not adequate for the degree of severity of the disease and do not always follow current guidelines. In Spain, the epidemiological study IBERPOC showed that only 21.8% of COPD patients had been previously diagnosed.

General practitioners do not usually perform spirometry, and absence of spirometric determinations results in inadequate treatment and thus disease progression. When chronic airflow obstruction is unnoticed in individuals attending their physicians because of chronic respiratory symptoms, appropriate measures and/or smoking cessation treatment may not be indicated. The lack of spirometry may contribute to the confusion between the diagnosis of asthma and COPD, which has important implications in the patient's management and prognosis.

Main causes of delayed COPD diagnosis

- Symptoms not significant until COPD is well established
- Current smoker, not willing to quit
- Lack of acknowledge of disease characteristics and treatment
- Unavailability of spirometry in primary care

Delay in diagnosis implies an advanced deterioration of quality of life and pulmonary function due to the progressive natural history of the disease

Clinical features characteristic of COPD

- Chronic cough. Usually cough is productive and mainly in the morning. Cough is not related to severity of lung function impairment
- Expectoration. The characteristics of sputum are a good diagnostic tool in clinical practice. Infection is suspected when an increase in volume and/or purulence is present. If sputum volume is higher than 30 ml/day, bronchiectasis must be suspected
- Dyspnoea appears when a moderate or severe airflow obstruction is present and it is usually progressive

The clinical features of COPD appear around 45 or 50 years of age. Symptoms develop after a minimum exposure of 20 pack-years in susceptible individuals. Dyspnoea on exertion usually appears 10 years after the beginning of initial respiratory symptoms.

Up to 70% of COPD patients remain undiagnosed, thus receiving no treatment or smoking cessation therapy. Suspecting the diagnosis in current or

# 3 (ii) The problem of underdiagnosis

former smokers with chronic respiratory symptoms is crucial and performing spirometry in this population has a great diagnostic yield. Several studies have demonstrated the feasibility of COPD screening in general practice.

## COPD screening criteria

- Older than 55 years
- Current or former smokers for more than 30 years
- Chronic cough and phlegm or chronic wheezing

** If all three criteria are present, probability of COPD is 45%*

# Initial evaluation

# 4

COPD should be suspected in every individual with a tobacco exposure of 10 pack-years or more, and older than 40 years of age.

## Diagnosis and initial assessment

- Forced spirometry showing CAFL
  FEV1<80% and FEV1/FVC<70%
- BDT
- Exclusion of other causes of CAFL (chronic asthma and bronchiectasis)
- Chest X-ray
- Additional:
  - serum AAT determination
  - arterial gasometry
  - EKG

CAFL: chronic airway flow limitation; BDT: bronchodilator test; AAT: alpha-1 antitrypsin

# 5 (i) Follow-up

## Factors to be considered during COPD follow-up

- General issues
  - health education, smoking cessation advice, diet and exercise, vaccination
  - family and psycho-social parameters
- Clinical evaluation
  - symptoms, treatment optimization, exacerbations
- Additional tests
  - haemogram: detection of polyglobulia
  - EKG and echocardiography: cor pulmonale
  - X-ray: detection of COPD derivated complications (pneumonia, pneumothorax) and/or associated diseases (lung cancer, heart failure, cor pulmonale)
- Detection of respiratory failure (RF)
  - acute RF: gasometry is mandatory
  - chronic RF: gasometry is suitable for the diagnosis and prescription of LTOT
  - pulsioximetry
  - exacerbation assessment
  - hypoxemia on exertion (exercise test)
  - chronic respiratory failure follow-up
- Treatment compliance evaluation
  - consider associations of different drugs in the same inhalation device
  - compliance with treatment
  - review of inhalation skills

LTOT: long term oxygen therapy

# Follow-up

5 (ii)

## Scheduled visits

| | Mild COPD | Moderate COPD | Severe COPD |
|---|---|---|---|
| Scheduled visit | annual | 6–12 months | 3 months |
| Spirometry | annual | 6–12 months | 6 months |
| Gasometry | — | 12 months | 6–12 months |
| EKG | — | annual | 12 months |

# 6(i) Spirometry

Spirometry is the best standardized and most reproducible diagnostic test for COPD and should be performed on every individual with suspected COPD. The spirometer is an essential tool for suitable management of respiratory patients in general practice, but several conditions are required to warranty quality in technique in order to obtain reliable results.

Detection of airflow limitation, particularly at the beginning of the disease, and an initial evaluation of treatment response can be detected by spirometric measurements. FEV1 is defined as forced expiratory volume during the first second and it is the best parameter related to life expectancy, exercise tolerance and surgery risk of these patients. Forced vital capacity (FVC) is the total expirated volume during a forced manoeuvre. Airflow obstruction exists when FEV1 is below 80% predicted and FEV1/FVC is below 70%. FEV1/FVC is a useful parameter to follow-up in mild and moderate cases. FEV1 is recommended for following-up the patients during the progression of the disease—FVC decreases faster than FEV1 so the relation between them tends to balance, creating a false perception of stabilization. Spirometry is not readily available for most GPs; in Spain, only 35–45% of GPs request pulmonary function tests in patients with obstructive lung disease.

## Bronchodilator test assessment

- To distinguish between asthma and COPD: if FEV1 becomes normal after bronchodilator administration probable diagnosis is asthma
- To establish the best FEV1 for a patient
- To determine prognosis of the disease: bronchodilation response is inversely related to FEV1 decline
- To evaluate the potential response to treatment

# Spirometry

6 (ii)

## Preparation for forced spirometry

- Periodical calibration is recommended
- Training of technician is mandatory
- Patient must be instructed about the manoeuvre procedure in order to get a maximum effort
- Comfortable dress is recommended
- Cessation of caffeine intake during previous hours is also recommended
- Bronchodilator treatment is not allowed during previous hours

## Forced spirometry manoeuvre

- Manoeuvre must be explained clearly to the patient
- Patient should be seated
- Nose occluded with a nose-clip
- A maximum inspiration followed by a forced expiration should be performed. Expiration beginning has to be rapid and intensive and continuous till airflow drops near zero (expiratory time >6 s)
- Three reproducible manoeuvres are required (FEV1 and FVC must not vary >5% or >100 ml)

# 6(iii) Spirometry

## Forced spirometry evaluation

- Obtained results have to be compared with reference values according to age, height, weight, sex and race
- Airflow obstruction not completely reversible is confirmed by the determination of FEV1 <80% predicted after administration of a bronchodilator drug and FEV1/FVC <70%
- A good predictor of initial development of disease is the existence of FEV1≥80% predicted and FEV1/FVC<70%

# Algorithm for COPD diagnosis

7 (i)

The algorithm shown in Figure 1 is a proposal for COPD diagnosis process after disease is suspected due to clinical symptoms and tobacco exposure. If COPD is suspected (chronic tobacco exposure with clinical symptoms), diagnosis should be confirmed by a forced spirometry. Different scientific society quality criteria must be considered in each spirometry.

## COPD initial assessment

- Clinical evaluation: symptoms, clinical signs, tobacco exposure, comorbility, exacerbations, hospital admissions, nutritional status
- Forced spirometry and bronchodilator test
- Chest X-ray, arterial gasometry, seric alpha-1 antitrypsin determination, blood and urine tests, EKG, lung diffusing capacity test (DLCO) and pletismography volumes
- Initial treatment plan
- Education: information about disease, inhalation technique, tobacco advice, diet and exercise, influenza and pneumococcal vaccinations
- Quality of life evaluation
- Psychosocial evaluation

## COPD additional tests

- Haemogram: diagnosis of associated anaemia or polyglobulia
- Electrocardiography: assessment of ischaemic cardiopathy or right ventricular hypertrophy
- Seric alpha-1 antitrypsin determination at least once (WHO recommendation) for its prognosis value, substitutive treatment administration assessment, family evaluation and genetic advice

7 (ii)

# Algorithm for COPD diagnosis

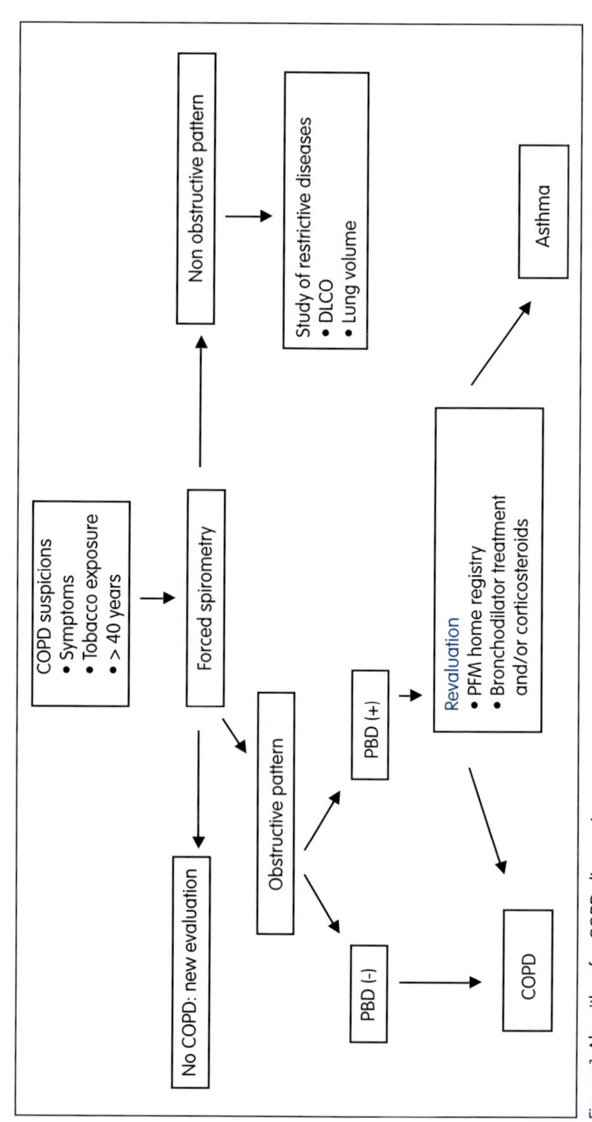


Figure 1 Algorithm for COPD diagnosis

# Algorithm for COPD diagnosis

7 (ii)

## COPD optional tests

- CO diffusion
- Pletismography
- Compliance assessment
- Walking test
- Respiratory ergometry
- Night oximetry
- Night polysomnography
- Thoracic computed tomography
- Echocardiography
- Lung haemodynamic evaluation

# 8 Classification of severity

Airflow obstruction is the main change in COPD. Measurement of FEV1, as percent predicted, is the best parameter for severity assessment. Several severity classifications are available, for example GOLD (Global Initiative for Chronic Obstructive Lung Disease).

## Severity classification of COPD (GOLD Guidelines)

| **Stage 0: at risk** | • Normal spirometric parameters<br>• Cough and/or sputum production |
|---|---|
| **Stage I: mild COPD** | • FEV1/FVC<70%<br>• FEV1 >80% predicted with or without chronic symptoms |
| **Stage II: moderate COPD** | • FEV1/FVC<70%<br>• FEV1 30–80% predicted<br>(IIA: FEV1 50–80% predicted)<br>(IIB: FEV1 30–50% predicted)<br>with or without chronic symptoms |
| **Stage III: severe COPD** | • FEV1/FVC<70%<br>• FEV1 <30% predicted or FEV1<50% and respiratory insufficiency or right heart failure |

# Causes of COPD

9 (i)

## Tobacco smoking

The most important risk factor for COPD is cigarette smoking. Pipe, cigar and other types of tobacco smoking popular in many countries are also risk factors for COPD. Cigarette smoke is a heterogeneous aerosol produced by incomplete combustion of the tobacco leaf. More than 4000 substances have been identified, including some that are pharmacologically active, antigenic, cytotoxic, mutagenic and carcinogenic as carbon monoxide, oxides of nitrogen, aromatic hydrocarbons, and nitrosamines. Some of the constituents of tobacco smoke are irritants, other induce toxic effects on the airway epithelium, causing cell damage or death as well as local inflammation. Oxidants in cigarette smoke have been shown to result in a protease/antiprotease imbalance in favour of proteolytic activity inducing tissue damage and parenchyma destruction with development of emphysema.

Smokers with COPD have higher tobacco consumption, greater dependence on nicotine and more than one-third have never tried to stop smoking. These figures indicate that the problem of COPD will continue to grow. A wealth of evidence suggests that obstructive respiratory diseases have become more common worldwide in the last century. The most important causal factor of COPD is active smoking, although only a proportion of smokers develop COPD therefore research is focusing on which endogenous factors predispose smokers to COPD. Diagnosis of COPD is questioned when tobacco exposure doesn't exist. Nevertheless only 15–20% of smokers develop the disease. That suggests that some other factors of individual susceptibility to tobacco smoke must exist.

Passive exposure to cigarette smoke also contributes to respiratory symptoms and COPD. This risk is especially relevant for children, and it is suggested that children of smokers show lower respiratory parameter data than children of non-smoking parents, and the incidence of respiratory tract infections and respiratory symptoms are more frequent too. Respiratory infections in early childhood are associated with reduced lung function and increased respiratory symptoms in adulthood. Airway hyper-responsiveness may also develop after exposure to tobacco smoke or other environmental insults and thus may be a result of smoking-related airway disease but how it influences the development of COPD is unknown.

### Air pollutants

There is evidence that air pollution is a major environmental risk factor for the beginning and/or the exacerbation of chronic respiratory conditions. Exposure to air pollutants can lead to an increase not only in morbidity but also in the mortality rate as well as increasing the number of admissions of patients with respiratory symptoms.

# 9 (ii) Causes of COPD

## Alpha-1 antitrypsin deficiency

Alpha-1 antitrypsin (AAT) deficiency is the first described genetic factor causing COPD. This protein is the main inhibitor of plasmatic proteases and its decreased plasmatic level contributes to development of emphysema. When protease inhibitors plasmatic levels are lower than protease levels, these non-inhibited enzymes cause lung parenchymal destruction and emphysema. Individuals with two Z alleles or one Z and one null allele, referred to as PIZ, have approximately 15% of normal plasma AAT levels. PIZ subjects who smoke cigarettes tend to develop more severe pulmonary impairment at an earlier age than non-smoking PIZ individuals. However, the development of COPD in PIZ subjects is not absolute. Due to its influence on COPD prognosis and prevention possibilities, the World Health Organization recommends AAT deficiency screening in all COPD patients. Other genes involved in the pathogenesis of COPD have not yet been identified but some (alpha-1 antichymotrypsin, alpha-2 microglobulin, extracellular superoxide dismutase) have been associated with COPD development.

## COPD aetiology

- Tobacco exposure is the main risk factor for developing COPD
- Passive tobacco exposure contributes to tobacco related diseases
- The role of other pollutants is not as well defined as cigarette smoking
- Alpha-1 antitrypsin deficiency is the first described genetic factor causing COPD

There is evidence that the risk of developing COPD is inversely related to socio-economic status. It is not clear, however, whether this pattern reflects occupational exposure to air pollutants, access to health facilities, poor nutrition or smoking habit.

# Smoking cessation

10(i)

Smoking status is believed to be a function of genetic and socio-demographic factors, environmental determinants, behavioural factors and specific dimensions of personality, in addition to the addiction to nicotine, with 70% of smokers reporting that they would like to quit. As with any drug addiction, social, economic, personal and political influences play a role in determining patterns of smoking prevalence and cessation. Since the most important risk factor for COPD is tobacco smoking, individuals who smoke should be encouraged to quit.

Smoking cessation is the single most effective and cost-effective intervention to reduce the risk of developing COPD and slow its progression. Smoking cessation is associated with improvement in respiratory parameters, reversal of the normal decline of FEV1, and significant decrease of respiratory symptoms such as cough and sputum production.

## Initial evaluation and smoking cessation follow-up

- Smoking status and processes of self-change (Prochaska and DiClemente): description of several states of smoking cessation process according which the current smoker gets ready to quit. These are: precontemplative, contemplutive, preparation to action
- Richmond's test: assessment of motivation to quit
- Measuring nicotine dependence (Fageström tolerance questionnaire): this simple questionnaire assesses degree of nicotine dependence and allows an accurate prescription of cessation treatment, mainly nicotine replacement therapy (NRT)
- Expired air carbon monoxide monitoring: tool to monitor tobacco abstinence

### Therapies for smoking cessation

Non-pharmacological management

- Minimal intervention: medical counselling, even a brief, 3 minute period of counselling in a clear, strong and personalized manner to urge a smoker to quit, can be effective and it is an available intervention for every health care worker
- Psychological management: smoking is considered the result of pharmacological and physiological factors, although behavioural items are important since the smoking habit results from a learning process reinforced by nicotine addiction. The physiological management has three thresholds, namely preparation to quit, cessation and maintenance of

# Smoking cessation

abstinence by preventing of relapse. Several approaches have been described and used with different and even contradictory results. Currently multicomponent programmes including cognitive and behavioural techniques plus specific relapse prevention therapy are recommended

- Progressive reduction: not entirely successful, easy to return to previous consumptions levels
- Others: mass media and community programmes, self-help programmes, educational materials, voluntary agencies, smoke-free environments, advertising bans and price increases can be effective measures

Pharmacotherapy is recommended when counselling is not enough to help patients to quit

- Nicotine replacement therapy (NRT): nicotine levels are progressively reduced during the quitting process, diminishing the absence symptoms. Administration route, dosage and timing have to be individually tailored, considering dependence grade, patterns of consumption and patient's characteristics. Combined NRT products are the most effective. NRT is not recommended when stroke, severe cardiac arrhythmia or gastrointestinal ulcer have recently occurred, generalized cutaneous diseases are present (only for patches) or during pregnancy and lactation.

Dosage, posology and side effects of nicotine replacement therapy

| Product | Posology | Adverse Event | Comments |
|---|---|---|---|
| Transdermal patch:<br>24 h: 30, 20, 10 mg<br>16 h: 15, 10, 5 mg | 1 patch/day | Cutaneous reactions | High safety and good tolerance |
| Chewing gum:<br>2 or 4 mg | Dosage and timing depending on dependence grade | Local reactions | High safety and good tolerance |
| Capsules 1 mg | Dosage and timing depending on dependence grade | Local reactions | High safety and good tolerance |
| Nasal spray | Dosage and timing depending on dependence grade | Local reactions | High safety and good tolerance |
| Others: sublingual tablet inhalator subcutaneous | Dosage and timing depending on dependence grade | Local reactions | High safety and good tolerance<br>Not available worldwide |

# Smoking cessation



- Bupropion: designed as an antidepressive drug, bupropion is the first non-nicotine related drug approved by Food and Drug Administration (FDA) for smoking cessation therapy. Its mechanism of action is not well known, but it works as a noradrenaline, dopamine and serotonin neuronal capture inhibitor. A role as a nicotine antagonist has been considered too. Bupropion controls abstinence symptoms, especially cravings and weight gain

Bupropion hydrochloride

| Posology | Adverse events | Comments |
|---|---|---|
| 150 mg/24 h, 1 week<br>150 mg/12 h, 7–9 weeks | Insomnia<br>Seizures<br>Cutaneous reactions | Contraindications: seizures, brain tumour, bipolar disorder, liver cirrhosis antecedents are present; alcohol abuse or quitting process; monoamine oxidase inhibitors (MAOI) treatment |

Other drugs used for smoking cessation

| | |
|---|---|
| Antidepressive | Fluoxetine<br>Moclobemide<br>Doxepin<br>Nortriptyline |
| CNS stimulant | Ephedrine<br>Caffeine<br>Methylfenidate |
| Anxiolytic | Buspirone<br>Ondansetron |
| Nicotine receptor blocker | Clonidine<br>Phenylpropanolamine |

# 11 (i) Pharmacological treatment of COPD

Treatment outcome is focused on improvement of patients' symptoms. Smoking cessation and long-term oxygen therapy, if chronic respiratory insufficiency is present, are the unique interventions that have proved to increase life expectancy.

## Objectives of treatment of COPD

- Smoking cessation
- Control of symptoms and prevention of exacerbations
- Preservation of lung function or decrease its impairment
- Improve quality of life and exertion tolerance
- Prevention or early detection and treatment of complications
- Side effects minimization
- Life expectancy improvement

Smoking cessation, vaccination and compliance with pharmacological treatment prescribed are essential for successful management. Drug treatment depends on severity of COPD and individualized tolerance and response. The principal drug families used in COPD management are: beta-2 adrenergics, anticholinergics, methylxanthines and inhaled or systemic corticosteroids.

# Pharmacological treatment of COPD

11 (ii)

## Stable COPD main thresholds treatment

- Smoking cessation
- Vaccination
- Pharmacological treatment:
  - bronchodilators:
    - short and long acting beta adrenergics
    - short and long acting anticholinergics
    - methylxanthines
  - anti-inflammatory drugs: corticosteroids (inhaled and systemic administration)
- Oxygen therapy
- Respiratory rehabilitation

### Vaccination

Every COPD patients must receive an influenza vaccination every year. Pneumococcal vaccination is also recommended.

### Bronchodilator treatment

Bronchodilators usually improve respiratory symptoms, although spirometric parameters may not change significantly. Inhaled administration is of choice.

# 11 (iii) Pharmacological treatment of COPD

## Dosage, posology and administration route of main inhaled bronchodilator drugs

| | Presentation | Minimum dosage/ frequency | Maximum dosage/ frequency | Onset of action | Max-imum effect | Length of action |
|---|---|---|---|---|---|---|
| **Beta-2 adrenergics:** | | | | | | |
| Salbutamol | ICP: 100 µg/inh | 200 µg/ 4–6 h | 1600 µg/day | 40–50 s | 15–20 min | 3–6 h |
| Terbutaline | ICP: 250 µg/inh<br>TH: 500 µg/inh | 500 µg/ 4–6 h | 6000 µg/day | 40–50 s | 15–20 min | 3–6 h |
| Salmeterol | ICP: 25 µg/inh<br>AH: 50 µg/inh | 50 µg/ 12 h | 200 µg/day | 18 min | 3–4 h | 12 h |
| Formoterol | ICP: 12.5 µg/inh<br>TH: 9.0 µg/inh<br>AL: 12.5 µg/inh | 12.5 µg/ 12 h | 48 µg/day | 1–3 min | 2 h | 12 h |
| **Anticholinergics:** | | | | | | |
| Ipratropium bromide | ICP: 20 µg/inh<br>CI: 40 µg/inh | 20–40µg/ 6–8 h | 320 µg/day | 15 min | 30–60 min | 4–8 h |
| Tiotropium bromide | HA: 18 µg/inh | 18µg/day | 18µg/day | 30 min | 3 h | 24 h |
| **Methylxanthines:** | | | | | | |
| Theophylline | po: 100 mg<br>200 mg<br>300 mg<br>Retard<br>600 mg | po: 5–7 mg/kg/day | po: 12 mg/kg/day | 3 h | 6 h | 12 h |
| Aminophylline | iv: 5.6 mg/kg (in 20 min) | 0.6 mg/kg/h | 0.6 mg/kg/h | 20 min | 3 h | 6 h |

ICP: pressurized cartridge; inh: inhalation; TH: Turbuhaler; HA: HandiHaler; AH: Accuhaler; AL: Aerolizer; CI: inhaled tablets; po: by mouth; h: hours; min: minutes; s: seconds; iv: intravenous.

# Pharmacological treatment of COPD

# 11 (iv)

## Beta-2 adrenergics (short acting)

On appearance, or increase in, symptoms. These drugs are recommended on demand (rescue medication) both in stable phase or during exacerbations.

## Beta-2 adrenergics (long acting)

Twice daily administration improves treatment compliance. Recent studies have shown an improvement in quality of life using 50 μg/12 hours of salmeterol.

Indications for long action beta-2 adrenergics

- Night symptoms
- Permanent symptom relief
- Decrease of daily inhalations

## Anticholinergics (short and long acting)

The main objective of this group is maintenance treatment of symptomatic stable COPD. Recently, tiotropium bromide has been launched; its main characteristic is its long half-life that allows once-daily administration. Patients usually experience a decrease in frequency of exacerbations and hospital admissions.

## Methylxanthines

The beneficial effects of this group of drugs include bronchodilation, increase of diuresis, improvement of diaphragmatic function and protection against muscle fatigue. However, they have a narrow therapeutic margin (between 10–20 μg/dl of plasma levels).

Most relevant indication of theophylline is optimizing bronchodilator effects of other groups such as anticholinergics and beta-2 adrenergics. Increasing the drug dosage increases the risk of toxic event.

# Pharmacological treatment of COPD

Factors influencing serum theophylline levels

| Increase concentrations: | Decrease concentrations: |
|---|---|
| Advanced age | Current smoker |
| Concomitant diseases:<br>• Heart failure<br>• Liver disease<br>• Hypoxia | Hypoproteic diet |
| Drugs:<br>• Cimetidine<br>• Allopurinol<br>• Ciprofloxacin<br>• Contraceptive<br>• Erythromycin | Enzymatic inductor drugs:<br>• Barbiturates<br>• Benzodiazepine<br>• Rifampicin<br>• Isoniazid |

## Anti-inflammatory treatment

### Oral corticosteroids and COPD

Oral corticosteroids are recommended for respiratory exacerbations with a dosage of 0.5 mg/kg for 7 to 15 days.

### Inhaled corticosteroids

These are used in clinical daily practice, although its recommendation is controversial. Advantages include: decrease of respiratory symptoms, improvement in quality of life, reduction in number of severe exacerbations and hospital admission in patients with moderate to severe disease (FEV1<50% predicted).

Nevertheless, some disadvantages exist: high cost, absence of improvement of spirometric parameters in most patients and side effects in long-term administration.

Another treatment option is the administration of an inhaled corticosteroid and a long acting beta-2 adrenergic through the same inhalation device. There are two variants of this treatment, both administered as dry powder: fluticasone propionate and salmeterol via Accuhaler and budesonide and formoterol via Turbuhaler.

Clinical trials have demonstrated that combination treatment has an additive bronchodilator effect and prevents exacerbations, particularly in severe COPD patients.

# Pharmacological treatment of COPD

11 (vi)

The bronchodilator effect of the combination, measured by the FEV1 both at peak (1–3 hours after administration) and at trough (before administration of the next dose) concentrations is of a higher magnitude in COPD patients with positive bronchodilator test results. In contrast, tiotropium bromide, a once daily, long acting anticholinergic, has a superior bronchodilator effect than the combination treatment in COPD patients with negative bronchodilator test results.

At present, there is no evidence of a therapeutic benefit resulting from the use of tiotropium together with a long acting beta-2 adrenergic and/or an inhaled corticosteroid.

Indications of inhaled corticosteroids

- Severe COPD (FEV1<50% predicted)
- Frequent exacerbations
- Accelerated impairment of lung function
- Improvement of symptoms or significant increase of exertion tolerance after oral corticosteroid administration

Inhaled corticosteroids not recommended

- Mild COPD
- Non atopic signs
- Negative bronchodilator test
- Absence of response after oral corticosteroid administration

# 11 (vii) Pharmacological treatment of COPD

## Adverse effects of COPD treatment

| | Side effects | Comments |
|---|---|---|
| Beta-2 adrenergics | Cough, oropharyngeal discomfort | Caution MAOI and TAD co-administration |
| | Bronchoconstriction | Antagonism with beta-blockers (salmeterol) |
| | Palpitations, tachycardia | Caution MAOI and TAD co-administration |
| | Tremor | Tachyphylaxis (except associated with inhaled corticoids) |
| | Hypokalaemia | |
| | Nausea, vomiting | |
| Anticholinergics | Dry mouth<br>Paradoxical bronchoconstriction | Contraindicated if hypersensitivity to atropine is present |
| Methylxanthines | Nausea, vomiting | Arrhythmia<br>Seizures |
| | Insomnia, headache | |
| Corticoids | Overweight, muscle weakness myopathy | |
| | Diabetes, Osteoporosis | |
| | Gastric and ophthalmic injury | |
| | Cutaneous and capillary fragility | |
| | Psychiatric alterations | |

MAOI: monoamine oxidase inhibitors; TAD: tricyclic antidepressants

## Stepwise treatment

Smoking cessation advice, influenza and pneumococcal vaccination and recommendation about regular exertion is mandatory.

# Pharmacological treatment of COPD

11 (viii)

## Proposal of treatment (mild and moderate COPD)

- Paucisymptomatic patients:
  - Ipratropium bromide or inhaled beta-2 adrenergic
- Symptomatic patients:
  - Inhaled long action anticholinergics or inhaled long action beta-2 adrenergics
  - Association of both
  - Add theophyllines (discontinue if effectiveness is not observed)
  - Inhaled corticosteroids should be considered

## Proposal of treatment (severe COPD)

- Inhaled corticosteroids should be added when previous bronchodilators failed to control symptoms
- Consider combined therapy: inhaled corticosteroid plus long-acting beta-2 adrenergic, especially if the patient has a positive bronchodilator test
- A rehabilitation programme should be considered
- Long term oxygen therapy is indicated if hypoxemic
- Lung volume reduction surgery should be considered in advanced emphysema
- Lung transplantation should be offered when <65 years of age

## Oxygen therapy

It is well known that oxygen improves life expectancy of COPD patients who suffer from chronic respiratory insufficiency. To be effective, minimum administration of 16 hours per day is required.

# 11 (ix) Pharmacological treatment of COPD

## Long term oxygen therapy indication

- $PaO_2$ <55 mmHg
- $PaO_2$ below 55–60 mmHg and one of following criteria:
  - polyglobulia
  - pulmonary hypertension
  - clinical or electrocardiographic signs of chronic right heart failure
  - impairment of intellectual functions
  - arrhythmia or heart failure

## Inhalation devices

### Advantages of inhaled therapy

- Better distribution of drug in the airways
- Localized and direct action
- Faster speed of action
- Lower doses
- Identical efficacy than that obtained by parenteral administration
- Less adverse effects than observed at other dosage (specially parenteral administration)
- Comfortable for transporting and utilization
- Favourable cost/benefit rate

# Pharmacological treatment of COPD

11 (x)

## Metered-dose inhalers (MDI)

### Pressurized cartridge

The main characteristic is generating particles between 2 and 4 microns, which can reach the distal airways. The body of the inhaler is a metallic cartridge in which the active drug is in solution together with the propellant gas (chlorofluorocarbons). A valve releases a controlled dose puff.

### Autohaler systems

Inhalation dispenser with an inspiration-activated device. Similar to the conventional pressurized cartridge, instead of a valve system it dispenses aerosol simultaneously with the patient's inspiration.

### Inhalation chambers

Inhalation chambers are designed to improve efficacy of pressurized cartridges and reduce oropharyngeal deposition of the inhaled medication. The evaporation of the propellant (freon) induces a decrease in particle size and allows the deposition in peripheral airways.

## Dry powder inhalers

The difficulties in adequate use of MDI, as well as concerns about the use of propellants such as freon, have favoured the development of new dry powder inhalers. Bronchodilators and anti-inflammatory drugs are available with such presentations.

Principal characteristics of dry powder inhalers

- Generation of particles in the range 1–2 microns
- Known, exact and repetitive dosing
- Ideal inspiratory flow for correct inhalation between 30 and 60 L/min
- No propellant gases are used

# 11 (xi) Pharmacological treatment of COPD

## Turbuhaler

This is a cylindrical device with a reservoir for the drug (micronized dry powder). Particle size generated is 1 micron. Inhalation induces a high speed flow due to turbulence production in the helicoidal tubes. Up to 200 doses can be dispensed.

## Accuhaler

Each measured dose is either contained in a capsule or a disc, which is then ruptured by the device, before inhalation. The capsules and discs have to be carefully stored so that the powder does not become damp or the capsules too brittle.

## HandiHaler

A dry powder inhaler device. To activate the device, patients place a single capsule in the mechanism, press a button to puncture the capsule, and then inhale slowly.

## Main characteristics of the different devices

| Device | Advantages | Disadvantages |
|---|---|---|
| Pressurized cartridge | Easy procedure<br>Activation by minimum inspiratory flux<br>Rapid action<br>Cheap and comfortable<br>Local and non-systemic effects<br>Known, exact and repetitive dose | Difficult procedure (40% of patients perform the wrong technique)<br>High oropharyngeal deposition<br>Chlorofluorocarbons can cause bronchospasm |
| Autohaler | Coordination trigger-inspiration is not required<br>Low inspiratory flux activation (between 18 and 30 L/min)<br>Easy for children and the elderly to use | |
| Inhalation chambers | Reduce the incidence of oral candidiasis after corticosteroid administration<br>Improved bronchial distribution of inhaled medication | Bulky and difficult to handle<br>Not adjustable to some dry powder inhalers |

# Non-pharmacological treatment

12 (i)

## Rehabilitation

The goals of pulmonary rehabilitation are to reduce symptoms, improve quality of life, and increase participation in everyday activities. Those objectives must be pursued through a healthy living style, good self-management of pharmacotherapy, respiratory muscles training and decrease of dyspnoea perception. Every COPD patient benefits from exercise training programmes, with improvements in exercise tolerance and dyspnoea.

Tools for initial evaluation in a rehabilitation programme:

- Quality of life questionnaires: Chronic Respiratory Disease Questionnaire (CRQ), St. George's Respiratory Questionnaire (SGRQ)
- Evaluation of exercise tolerance: Six minute walking test, shuttle walking test
- Evaluation of dyspnoea: Medical Research Council (MRC) scale, Mahler index (BDI/TDI), Borg index

### Exercise training

Exercise training improves ventilatory mechanics and gas exchange. Specific exercises for upper limbs facilitate daily activities. These strategies are not standardized but are supported by studies that showed improvement of the main limiting symptoms of COPD, particularly dyspnoea on exertion. The controlled breathing techniques produce an increase of tidal volume, decrease of respiratory frequency and improve the efficacy of respiratory muscles. Training of the respiratory muscles optimizes the energy consumption and oxygen use by improvement of thoracic dynamics.

### Respiratory physiotherapy

Respiratory physiotherapy facilitates drainage of respiratory secretions, inducing a decrease of resistance to airflow and possibly preventing infection and favouring patient's comfort.

### Nutrition counselling

There is increasing evidence of the deleterious effect of malnutrition on progression of lung function impairment and quality of life, together with an increase in mortality and mobility associated with low body mass index. Malnutrition is an independent factor of poor prognosis in COPD. Causes of malnutrition in COPD are not well established, but the primary postulated mechanism is hypermetabolism resulting in elevated total caloric expenditure arising from increased airway resistance, increased $O_2$ cost of ventilation, increased dietary induced thermogenesis, inefficient substrate use and, perhaps, increased levels of proinflammatory cytokines.

# 12(ii) Non-pharmacological treatment

## Education

A healthy way of living includes smoking avoidance, regular exercise and adequate diet. Education about the effects of the different drugs used for pulmonary disease and training on use of inhalers is an important aspect to optimize the compliance and effectiveness of COPD treatment.

## Surgical treatments

### Lung volume reduction surgery (LVRS)

The lung volume reduction surgery is a therapeutic option for patients affected by severe and heterogeneous emphysema.

Inclusion criteria for LVRS

- Severe airway obstruction with forced expiratory volume within the first second (FEV1) decreased to less than 35% of individual normal baseline function
- Severe pulmonary hyperinflation and air trapping with a total lung capacity (TLC) of more than 125% of normal pulmonary function as assessed by whole-body plethysmograph, combined with a residual volume (RV) increase to more than 200% of the individual predicted value
- Radiologically identified (CT) regionally heterogeneous high-degree emphysema of the lung, where target areas without function (perfusion scan) can be outlined and easily excised

Exclusion criteria for LVRS

- Age >75 years
- $PaO_2$ at rest (FiO2 0.21): <50 mmHg
- $PaCO_2$ at rest: >50 mmHg
- Mean pressure, pulmonary artery: >35 mmHg
- Pre-existing severe airway disease: asthma, fibrosis, bronchiectasis
- Treatment with steroids >20 mg prednisolone/day or equivalents
- Acute respiratory infection
- Pleural thickening due to previous infections/operations
- Severe disorders of the thoracic cavity causing restrictions: osteoporosis, scoliosis
- Severe concomitant disorders: high cardiovascular risk factor, progressive malignancies
- Homogeneous or lower lobe focused emphysema

There is currently not enough evidence to support the widespread use of lung volume reduction surgery, despite some encouraging reports. Several large-scale randomized studies are underway.

## Transplantation

The first lung transplantation was performed in 1963. The development of immunosuppressive therapy has produced improvements in survival. Lung transplantation has been shown to improve quality of life and functional capacity, thus it must be considered in carefully selected patients with severe COPD in whom other therapeutic alternatives have failed to control the symptoms.

# 12(iv) Non-pharmacological treatment

Inclusion criteria for lung transplantation

- Life expectancy because of lung disease <2 years
- Not older than 55–60 years old
- FEV1<35% predicted
- Hypercapnoea
- Existence of secondary pulmonary hypertension

Exclusion criteria for lung transplantation

- Non controlled infection
- Malignancy
- Existence of other life-threatening diseases, especially severe left ventricle dysfunction, or psychiatric conditions presupposed to avoid post-transplantation treatment compliance
- Current smoker

## Conclusions

1. Every COPD patient can benefit from exercise training programmes with improvements in exercise tolerance and dyspnoea.

2. There is currently no sufficient evidence that would support the widespread use of lung volume reduction surgery.

3. Lung transplantation may be considered in carefully selected patients with severe COPD.

# Acute exacerbations

13(i)

## Definition

The chronic and progressive course of COPD is often aggravated by short periods of increasing symptoms, particularly increasing cough, dyspnoea and production of sputum, which can become purulent. These episodes are known as acute exacerbations or simply exacerbations of COPD. Definition of such events is difficult and no standard clinical diagnostic criteria exist, although the combination of symptoms described by Anthonisen and co-workers have been widely used: increased dyspnoea and increased production or purulence of sputum. No diagnostic test is available for diagnosing exacerbations.

## Incidence and importance

Patients with moderate COPD suffer from a mean of two exacerbations per year (mean FEV1=50–55% predicted), but this number is dependent on the degree of functional impairment at baseline. Patients with more advanced disease may suffer from an increasing number of episodes. Acute exacerbations are the most frequent cause of medical visits, hospital admissions and death among patients with chronic lung disease.

Failure rate of ambulatory treatment of exacerbations of COPD ranges from 12% to 26%. Identification of risk factors for failure of ambulatory treatment may permit the implementation of more aggressive broad-spectrum treatment and closer follow-up.

### Risk factors for failure after ambulatory treatment of exacerbation of COPD

- Coexisting cardiopulmonary disease
- Increasing number of previous visits to the GP for respiratory problems (>3/year)
- Increasing number of previous exacerbations (>3/year)
- Increasing baseline dyspnoea
- Severity of FEV1 impairment (FEV1<35% predicted)
- Use of home oxygen
- Inadequate antibiotic therapy

# 13 (ii) Acute exacerbations

Failure of treatment may lead to hospital admission. The mortality of patients admitted to hospital with COPD exacerbation is about 10–14%, and mortality of those admitted to an intensive care unit (ICU) for exacerbations may be as high as 24%. Hospitalization has an important impact in COPD patients. After first admission to hospital, mean survival time has been estimated at 5.7 years, with COPD together with lung cancer being the main cause of death.

## Risk factors for hospitalization for exacerbation of COPD

- Significant comorbidities*
- Severity of FEV1 impairment (FEV1<35% predicted)
- High admission rate for previous exacerbations
- Advanced age (>70 years)

* Significant comorbidities are: insulin-dependent diabetes mellitus, cardiac insufficiency and ischaemic heart disease.

The mean total cost of an acute exacerbation of COPD was estimated to be $159 in a recent study in primary care in Spain, the main part being due to hospitalization which represented 58% of the total cost, followed by the total drug acquisition cost of 32.2%. Failure implies a cost that is three times higher than the cost of management of the exacerbation, particularly due to the high cost of hospitalization. If percentages of relapse could be reduced, especially in severe cases, valuable resources could be saved.

Frequent exacerbations have been demonstrated to have a negative impact on quality of life in patients with COPD. Therefore, identification of patients with increasing risk of frequent exacerbations is important for management of the disease.

# Acute exacerbations

13 (iii)

## Risk factors for frequent exacerbations of COPD (> 2 per year)

- Chronic bronchial mucus hypersecretion
- Severity of FEV1 impairment (FEV1<35% predicted)
- Frequent past exacerbations
- Advanced age (>70 years)
- Daily cough and wheeze

From the analysis of the three preceding tables it can be concluded that advanced COPD as measured by a low FEV1 is the main risk factor for poor outcome. Severity of the baseline disease is the best marker of risk.

## Aetiology

Aetiology of exacerbations is still a matter of controversy. Since respiratory secretions of some patients with stable COPD carry potentially pathogenic microorganisms in significant concentrations, the isolation of such microorganisms during exacerbations should not be interpreted as a definite demonstration of their pathogenic role. However, studies performed with specific invasive techniques have shown that both the number of patients with pathogenic bacteria in respiratory secretions, and their concentrations in bronchial secretions increase during exacerbations.

Up to three-quarters of exacerbations can be infectious in origin and bacteria are for responsible three-quarters of infective exacerbations. Today, the presence of green (purulent) sputum as opposed to white (mucus) is one of the best and easiest methods to predict bacterial aetiology and the need for antibiotic therapy.

# 13 (iv) Acute exacerbations

## Aetiology of acute exacerbations of COPD

Infectious exacerbations
(approximately 60–80% of all exacerbations)
Frequent (70–85% of all infectious exacerbations)
*Haemophilus influenzae*
*Streptococcus pneumoniae*
*Moraxella catarrhalis*
Viruses (influenza/parainfluenza, rhinoviruses, coronaviruses)

Infrequent (15–30% of all infectious exacerbations)
*Pseudomonas aeruginosa*
Opportunistic Gram negatives
*Staphylococcus aureus*
*Chlamydia pneumoniae*
*Mycoplasma pneumoniae*

Non-infectious exacerbations
(20–40% of all exacerbations)
Heart failure
Pulmonary embolism
Non-pulmonary infections
Pneumothorax

(adapted from Miravitlles et al 2001)

The degree of functional respiratory impairment of COPD patients indicates the presence of different microorganisms in the course of exacerbations. Individuals with severe pulmonary function impairment, manifested by FEV1<50% predicted, are at a six-fold greater risk of suffering acute exacerbations caused by *H. influenzae* or *P. aeruginosa* than patients presenting with FEV1>50%.

## Treatment: antibiotics

Bacterial infection is the main cause of acute exacerbations of COPD. There are other causes, however; no clear signs or symptoms allow us to differentiate between infectious and non-infectious exacerbations. Furthermore, clinical presentation of exacerbation is not characteristic of any particular microorganism, and no microbiologic diagnostic test is readily available for differential diagnosis. Thus, the decision on prescribing antibiotic therapy and the selection of antibiotic is made on an empirical basis.

Antibiotics have been shown to be superior to placebo in the treatment of exacerbations when at least two of the so-called Anthonisen criteria are present: increased dyspnoea, increased production of sputum and/or purulence of sputum. Recently, purulence of sputum has been demonstrated to be very sensitive and specific for the diagnosis of bacterial exacerbation and indicates the need for antibiotic therapy. Some guidelines recommend antibiotic therapy in all high-risk patients irrespective of the symptoms of exacerbation, since the risk of relapse or hospital admission is greater that the possibility of prescribing a course of antibiotics that may be unnecessary.

The antibiotic of choice will vary from country to country, based on prevalence of bacteria and, more importantly, differences in susceptibility to antibiotics of the causative bacteria. The reader is referred to local guidelines for the antibiotic of choice in their country.

## Factors influencing antibiotic choice for exacerbations of COPD

- Status of the patient
  - Bacteria isolated in previous exacerbations
  - Low FEV1 (<35%)
  - Number of courses of antibiotics the previous year
  - Colour of sputum
- Prevalent microorganisms
  - Beta-lactamase producing *H. influenzae*
  - Beta-lactamase producing *M. catarrhalis*
  - Penicillin-resistant *S. pneumoniae*
  - Macrolide-resistant *S. pneumoniae*

As an example, prevalence of macrolide-resistant *S. pneumoniae* in the UK in 2000 was 12.2%, but in France it was 58.1%. Production of beta-lactamase by *H. influenzae* was 13.9% in the UK and 33.1% in France in the same year.

There are a wide variety of antibiotics to choose for treatment of exacerbations of COPD. Guidelines recommend the use of so-called traditional

# 13 (vi) Acute exacerbations

antibiotics, such as amoxicillin or tetracycline in low-risk patients in countries with a low prevalence of antibiotic resistance, such as the Netherlands, UK and other North European countries. However, in countries with a high percentage of resistant strains or in patients with risk factors for treatment failure, antibiotic choice must consider amoxicillin/clavulanate, the new fluoroquinolones (moxifloxacin, gatifloxacin, levofloxacin), azithromycin or telithromycin.

Characteristics of the antibiotics most frequently used in ambulatory treatment of acute exacerbations of COPD:

| | Microbiological activity | | | Frequency | Duration (days) | AE |
|---|---|---|---|---|---|---|
| | *S. pneumo* | *H. flu* | *M. cat* | | | |
| Amoxicillin | +/– | +/– | – | tid | 7-10 | + |
| Tetracycline | + | + | + | bid/tid | 7-10 | ++ |
| Cefuroxime | +/– | + | + | bid | 7-10 | ++ |
| TMP/SMX | +/– | +/– | + | bid | 10-14 | ++ |
| Amoxi/clav | +/– | + | + | tid/bid | 7-10 | +++ |
| Clarithromycin | +/– | +/– | + | bid | 7-10 | ++ |
| Moxifloxacin | +++ | ++ | ++ | od | 5 | + |
| Levofloxacin | + | ++ | ++ | od | 7-10 | + |
| Telithromycin | +++ | + | ++ | od | 5 | ++ |
| Azythromycin | + | +/– | ++ | od | 5 | ++ |

*S. pneumo: Streptococcus pneumoniae; H. flu: Haemophilus influenzae; M. cat: Moraxella catarrhalis;* AE: adverse events

## Treatment: bronchodilators and corticosteroids

Acute exacerbations of COPD present with increasing dyspnoea in the majority of cases. Both infectious and non-infectious exacerbations are the result of an ongoing inflammatory reaction in the bronchial mucosa; therefore, anti-inflammatory and bronchodilator therapy are mandatory.

A short course of oral corticosteroids will accelerate recovery from exacerbations and reduce the rate of relapse in patients with moderate to severe COPD. Multiple different regimens have been proposed and no

# Acute exacerbations

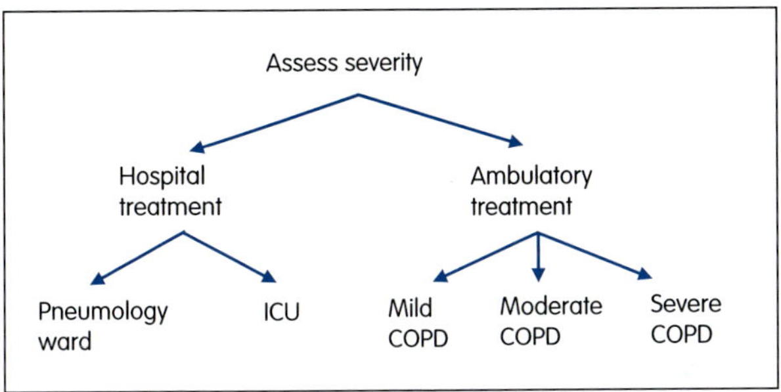


Figure 1 Assessment of severity of acute exacerbations of COPD. ICU: intensive care unit

standard regimen exists. Patients can be treated with 0.5 mg/kg/day of methylprednisolone or equivalent in a single morning dose for 7 to 14 days. Treatment for more than 14 days has not been demonstrated to be of more benefit and will increase the likelihood of adverse side effects.

Inhaled bronchodilators, particularly short acting, must be given at increased dose during exacerbations.

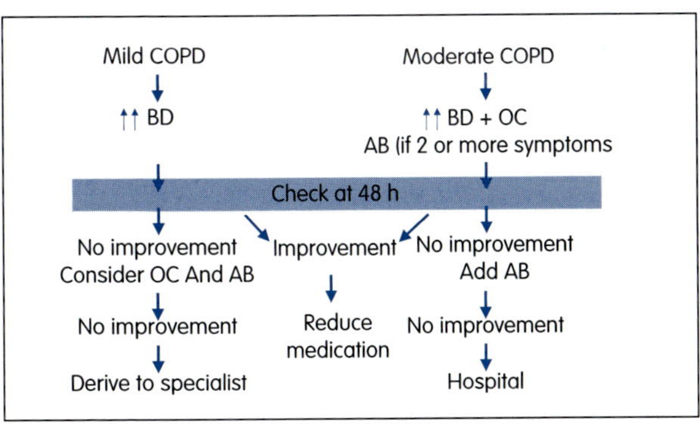


Figure 2 Treatment of mild and moderate acute exacerbations of COPD. BD: bronchodilators; AB: antibiotics; OC: oral corticosteroids.

# Acute exacerbations

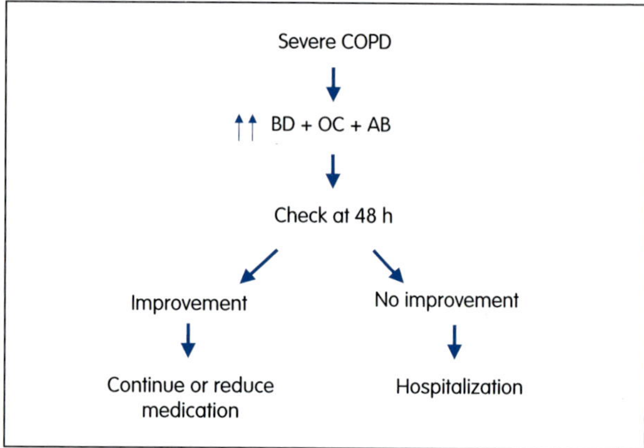


Figure 3 Treatment of severe acute exacerbation of COPD. BD: bronchodilators; AB: antibiotics; OC: oral corticosteroids.

# When to refer a COPD patient to hospital or a specialist

14 (i)

## Criteria for referral to pneumologist

- Scheduled visit
  - diagnosis or treatment doubts
  - non satisfying response to suitable treatment
  - long term oxygen therapy prescription
  - non invasive mechanical ventilation prescription
  - referral to LVRS or lung transplantation
  - emphysema occurred in patients younger than 45 years
  - moderate or severe COPD
  - sleep disorders
  - rehabilitation programme prescription
- Emergencies:
  - severe COPD exacerbation

## Indications for arterial gasometry

- FEV1 <1 litre
- Moderate or severe dyspnoea
- Pulmonary hypertension
- Haematocrit >55%
- Congestive heart failure
- Chronic cor pulmonale
- Cyanosis

# 14 (ii) When to refer a COPD patient to hospital or a specialist

## Factors suggesting good COPD management

- Maintenance of ideal weight and exercise
- Haematocrit <55%
- $PaO_2$>70 mmHg (stable phase)
- Influenza and pneumococcal vaccination
- Decrease in number or severity of exacerbations
- Right inhalation technique

# Bibliography

A clinical practice guideline for treating tobacco use and dependence: A US Public Health Service report. The Tobacco Use and Dependence Clinical Practice Guideline Panel, Staff, and Consortium Representatives.

Adams SG, Melo J, Luther M, Anzueto A. Antibiotics are associated with lower relapse rates in outpatients with acute exacerbations of COPD. Chest 2000; 117: 1345–1352.

Anthonisen NR, Manfreda J, Warren CPW, Hershfield ES, Harding GKM, Nelson NA. Antibiotic therapy in exacerbations of chronic obstructive pulmonary disease. Ann Intern Med 1987; 106: 196–204.

Anthonisen NR, Connett JE, Kiley JP et al. The Lung Health Study Research Group: effects of smoking intervention and the use of an inhaled anticholinergic bronchodilator on the rate of decline of $FEV_1$. JAMA 1994; 272: 1497–1505.

Ball P, Harris JM, Lowson D, Tillotson G, Wilson R. Acute infective exacerbations of chronic bronchitis. Q J Med 1995; 88: 61–68.

Balter MS, Hyland RH, Low DE, Renzi PM, Brade AC, Cole PJ. Recommendations on the management of chronic bronchitis. A practical guide for Canadian physicians. Can Med Ass J 1994; 151 (Suppl): 7–23.

Barnes PJ. Chronic Obstructive Pulmonary Disease. N Engl J Med 2000; 343: 269–280.

Brusasco V, Hodder R, Miravitlles M, Korducki L, Towse L, Kesten S. Health outcomes following treatment for six months with once daily tiotropium compared to twice daily salmeterol in patients with COPD. Thorax 2003; 58: 399–404.

Calverley P, Pawels R, Vestbo J et al. Combined salmeterol and fluticasone in the treatment of chronic obstructive pulmonary disease: a randomised controlled trial. Lancet 2003; 361: 449–456.

Celli BR, Snider GL, Heffner J et al. American Thoracic Society standards for the diagnosis and care of patients with chronic obstructive pulmonary disease. Am J Respir Crit Care Med 1995; 152: S77–S120.

Cerveri I, Accordini S, Verlato G et al. Variations in the prevalence across countries of chronic bronchitis and smoking habits in young adults. Eur Respir J 2001; 18: 85–92.

COPD Guidelines Group of the Standard of Care Committee of the British Thoracic Society (BTS). BTS Guidelines for the Management of Chronic Obstructive Pulmonary Disease. Thorax 1997; 52(Suppl): S1–S28.

Dal Negro R, Berto P, Tognella S, Quareni L, on behalf of GOLD Study Group. Cost-of-illness of lung disease in the TriVeneto Region, Italy: the GOLD Study. Monaldi Arch Dis Chest 2002; 57: 3–9.

Dickinson JA, Meaker M, Searle M et al. Screening older patients for obstructive airways disease in a semi-rural practice. Thorax 1999; 54: 501–505.

# Bibliography

Fageström KO. Measuring degree of physical dependence on tobacco smoking with references to individualization of treatment. Addict Behav 1978; 3: 235–241.

Fletcher C, Peto R. The natural history of chronic airflow obstruction. Br Med J 1977; 1(6077): 1645–1648.

Hilleman DE, Dewan N, Malesker M, Friedman M. Pharmacoeconomic evaluation of COPD. Chest 2000; 118: 1278–1285.

Hurd S. The impact of COPD on lung health worldwide. Epidemiology and incidence. Chest 2000; 117: 1S–4S.

Jacobson L, Hertzman P, Löfdahl CG et al. The economic impact of asthma and chronic obstructive pulmonary disease (COPD) in Sweden in 1980–1991. Respir Med 2000; 94: 247–255.

Jansson SA, Andersson F, Borg S, Ericsson A, Jonson E, Lundbäck B. Costs of COPD in Sweden according to disease severity. Chest 2002; 122: 1994–2002.

Jiménez CA, Masa F, Miravitlles M, Gabriel R, Viejo JL, Villasante C, Sobradillo V. Smoking characteristics: attitudes and dependence. Differences between healthy smokers and smokers with COPD. Chest 2001; 119: 1365–1370.

MacFarlane JT, Colville A, Guion A, MacFarlane RM, Rose DH. Prospective study of aetiology and outcome of adult lower respiratory tract infections in the community. Lancet 1993; 341: 511–514.

Mannino DM, Brown C, Giovino GA. Obstructive lung disease deaths in the United States from 1979 through 1993. An analysis using multiple-cause mortality data. Am J Respir Crit Care Med 1997; 156: 814–818.

Maurer JR, Frost AE, Estenne M, Higenbottam T, Glanville AR. International guidelines for the selection of lung transplant candidates. The International Society for Heart and Lung Transplantation, the American Society of Transplant physicians, the European Respiratory Society. Transplantation 1998; 66: 951–956.

Miravitlles M, Espinosa C, Fernández-Laso E, Martos JA, Maldonado JA, Gallego M and Study Group of Bacterial Infection in COPD. Relationship between bacterial flora in sputum and functional impairment in patients with acute exacerbations of COPD. Chest 1999; 116: 40–46.

Miravitlles M, Mayordomo C, Artés M, Sánchez Agudo L, Nicolau F, Segú JL on behalf of the EOLO group. Treatment of chronic obstructive pulmonary disease and its exacerbations in general practice. Respir Med 1999; 23: 173–179.

Miravitlles M, Fernández I, Guerrero T y Murio C. Desarrollo y resultados de un programa de cribado de la EPOC en Atención Primaria. El proyecto PADOC. Arch Bronconeumol 2000; 36: 500–505.

# Bibliography

Miravitlles M, Guerrero T, Mayordomo C, Sánchez-Agudo L, Nicolau F, Segú JL on Behalf of the EOLO Study Group. Factors associated with increased risk of exacerbation and hospital admission in a cohort of ambulatory COPD patients: a multiple logistic regression analysis. Respiration 2000; 67: 495–501.

Miravitlles M, Murio C, Guerrero T on Behalf of the DAFNE Study Group. Factors associated with relapse after ambulatory treatment of acute exacerbations of chronic bronchitis. A prospective multicenter study in the community. Eur Respir J 2001; 17: 928–933.

Miravitlles M. Epidemiology of chronic obstructive pulmonary disease exacerbations. Clin Pulm Med 2002; 9: 191–197

Miravitlles M. Exacerbations of chronic obstructive pulmonary disease: when are bacteria important? Eur Respir J 2002; 20 (Suppl 36): 9s–19s.

Miravitlles M, Murio C, Guerrero T, Gisbert R on behalf of the DAFNE study group. Pharmacoeconomic evaluation of acute exacerbations of chronic bronchitis and COPD. Chest 2002; 121: 1449–1455.

Miravitlles M, Murio C, Guerrero T, Gisbert R on behalf of the DAFNE study group. Costs of chronic bronchitis and COPD. A one year follow-up study. Chest 2003; 123: 784–791.

Monsó E, Ruiz J, Rosell A et al. Bacterial infection in chronic obstructive pulmonary disease. A study of stable and exacerbated outpatients using the protected specimen brush. Am J Respir Crit Care Med 1995; 152: 1316–1320.

Pauwels RA, Buist AS, Calverley PM, Jenkins CR, Hurd SS, GOLD Scientific Committee. Global strategy for the diagnosis, management, and prevention of chronic obstructive pulmonary disease. NHLBI/WHO Global Initiative for Chronic Obstructive Lung Disease (GOLD) Workshop summary. Am J Respir Crit Care Med 2001; 163: 1256–1276.

Prescott E, Lange P, Vestbo J and the Copenhagen City Heart Study Group. Socioeconomic status, lung function and admission to hospital for COPD: results from the Copenhagen City Heart Study. Eur Respir J 1999; 13: 1109–1114.

Prochaska J, DiClemente C. Stages and process of self-change of smoking towards an integrative model of change. J Consult Clin Psychol 1983; 51: 390–395.

Richmond RL, Kehoe L, Webster IW. Multivariate models for predicting abstention following intervention to stop smoking by general practitioner. Addiction 1993; 88: 1127–1135.

Rutten van Mölken MPMH, Postma MJ, Joore MA, Van Genugten MLL, Leidl R, Jager JC. Current and future medical costs of asthma and chronic obstructive pulmonary disease in the Netherlands. Respir Med 2000; 93: 779–787.

# Bibliography

Seemungal TAR, Donaldson GC, Paul EA, Bestall JC, Jeffries DJ, Wedzicha JA. Effect of exacerbation on quality of life in patients with chronic obstructive pulmonary disease. Am J Respir Crit Care Med 1998; 157: 1418–1422.

Siafakas NM, Vermeire P, Pride NB, Paoletti P, Gibson J, Howard P, Yernault JC, Decramer M, Higenbottam T, Postma DS et al. Optimal assessment and management of chronic obstructive pulmonary disease (COPD). The European Respiratory Society Task Force. Eur Respir J 1995; 8: 1398–1420.

Sobradillo V, Miravitlles M, Gabriel R, Jiménez-Ruiz CA, Villasante C, Masa JF, Viejo JL, Fernández-Fau L. Geographical variations in prevalence and underdiagnosis of COPD. Results of the IBERPOC multicentre epidemiological study. Chest 2000; 118: 981–989.

Sorlie PD, Kannel WB, O'Connor G. Mortality associated with respiratory function and symptoms in advanced age. The Framingham Study. Am Rev Respir Dis 1989; 140: 379–384.

Stang P, Lydick E, Silberman C, Kempel A, Keating ET. The prevalence of COPD. Using smoking rates to estimate disease frequency in the general population. Chest 1999; 117: 354s–359s.

Stockley RA, O'Brien C, Pye A, Hill SL. Relationship of sputum color to nature and outpatient management of acute exacerbations of COPD. Chest 2000; 117: 1638–1645.

Szafranski W, Cukier A, Ramirez A et al. Efficacy and safety of budesonide/formoterol in the management of chronic obstructive pulmonary disease. Eur Respir J 2003; 21: 74–81.

US Department of Health and Human Services. The health benefits of smoking cessation: A report of the Surgeon General, 1990. Rockville, MD: Dept. Of Health and Human Services, Public Health Service, Center for Disease Control, Center for Chronic Disease Prevention and Health Promotion, Office on Smoking and Health. DHHS Publication (CDC) 1990; 90–8416.

Wilson L, Devine EB, So K. Direct medical costs of chronic obstructive pulmonary disease: chronic bronchitis and emphysema. Respir Med 2000; 94: 204–213.